the yoga
of nutrition

Cover illustration: a crystal.

ISBN 0-911857-03-6

Published and Distributed by
PROSVETA U.S.A. P.O. Box 49614
Los Angeles, CA 90049-0614

Omraam Mikhaël Aïvanhov

the yoga
of nutrition

Translated from the French

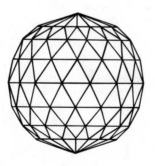

Collection Izvor
N° 204

EDITIONS 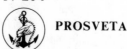 PROSVETA

By the same author:

(translated from the French)

Izvor Collection:

"Complete Works" Collection

CONTENTS

EDITOR'S NOTE

The reader is asked to bear in mind that the Editors have retained the spoken style of the Maître Omraam Mikhaël Aïvanhov in his presentation of the Teaching of the great Universal White Brotherhood, the essence of the Teaching being the spoken Word.

They also wish to clarify the point that the word *white* in Universal White Brotherhood, does not refer to colour or race, but to purity of soul. The Teaching shows how all men without exception (universal), can live a new form of life on earth (brotherhood), in harmony (white), and with respect for each other's race, creed and country... that is, Universal White Brotherhood.

1

NUTRITION CONCERNS THE WHOLE MAN

Today, I am going to talk on the subject of nutrition, dear brothers and sisters, and tell you things that are of the utmost importance. Very few, even amongst learned and highly evolved people, know these things. They may not seem interesting to you to start, but as you listen and especially as you practice these things, you will see that they are tremendously rich and rewarding, they can transform your entire existence.

Suppose that for one reason or another you are deprived of food for several days and are too feeble even to move. You may be erudite, you may be wealthy, but none of the things you know and none of the things you own, can equal the fruit or the piece of bread that you put into your mouth at that moment: one bite and you revive! One mouthful is all that is needed to make the forces and mechanisms of your entire system start working. There are certain elements in food that restore health and vigour more effectively than any thought, emotion, or will-power, but you do not realize this, food has little importance for you except as a means of satisfying your instincts and you do not believe it has any effect on you emotionally or intellectually. Yet food is what makes it possible for you to do everything you do, to talk and feel and think.

Initiates have always known the importance of nutrition, they discovered long ago that food is conceived and prepared in the divine laboratories above with infinite wisdom and that it contains magic elements that make it possible for man to receive revelations. They also know that they must create certain conditions before they can benefit from the food.

Although it is nutrition that is at the origin of wars and revolutions, it cannot be said that the world considers it of prime importance. Humans are instinctive about eating as are animals, and have no notion of the spiritual benefit to be derived from eating in a certain way... in fact they do not know how to eat. Watch people, you will see how mechanically and unconsciously they eat, swallowing without chewing and permitting all kinds of chaotic ideas and feelings to interfere with the process of digestion, the secreting and eliminating of poisons. And then they wonder why they fall ill: it is their way of eating. In families, everyone is busy reading, watching television, working... until they sit down to dinner... and then they start chattering, arguing, fighting. A meal eaten under such conditions makes you want to do nothing afterwards but sleep, you are so heavy and weighed down that you have no enthusiasm for anything. If you eat as you should, you feel fit, lucid of mind and ready to work after meals.

"Well, then how should one eat?" you ask. I will tell you what an Initiate does. First of all, knowing that he must prepare the best possible conditions in order to benefit from the elements Nature has prepared, he begins by recollecting himself, remaining silent and devoting his thoughts to his Creator (silence during meals is not the sole property of convents and monasteries, Initiates and sages have always eaten in silence). He knows also that the first mouthful is most important (the most important moment of any action is the first step) for it signals the release of forces which once released do not stop but continue to the end: if you begin in a state of harmony, whatever you do will be harmonious to the end.

And then he eats slowly and chews the food thoroughly, not only for the sake of his digestion, but because the mouth is a spiritual laboratory which absorbs the subtle etheric energies before sending the grosser particles on down to the stomach. The mouth is to the subtle planes what the stomach is to the physical plane, a highly perfected instrument with glands on and under the tongue that capture the etheric particles... which explains why you can be completely restored and cheered when you are weary and weak with hunger by the first mouthful *before* it has time to reach the stomach! The mouth distils energy and sends it to the nervous system before the less subtle elements can reach the stomach.

It should not surprise you to hear that etheric elements can be extracted from the food. Fruit for instance, is made of solid, liquid, gaseous and etheric matter: everybody is aware of the solid and liquid substance, but few are aware of the subtle aroma which belongs to the region of air. No one pays the slightest attention to the etheric side, which has to do with the colour and especially with the life of the fruit and which is the most important part of all, because it is these etheric particles that nourish our more subtle bodies....

Since beside his physical body man has other, more subtle bodies (the etheric, astral, mental, causal, buddhic and atmic bodies which are the seat of his psychic and spiritual functions), he might well wonder how to feed them rather than letting them starve. Man knows approximately what to feed his physical body (I say approximately because most people eat meat, which is bad for them both physically and psychically) but he has no idea what to give his etheric (vital) body, his astral (emotional) body, his mental body, to say nothing of the still higher bodies.

As I told you, it is an aid to the physical body to masticate thoroughly, but for the etheric body you need to add something more: respiration. In the same way that a breeze animates the flame (you blow on a spark to light a fire), so breathing deeply during the course of a meal makes for better combustion. Digestion, respiration and reflection are all forms of combustion, the only difference being in the degree of heat and the purity of the substance. If you stop eating from time to time and take a deep breath, the combustion that takes place allows the etheric body to extract the subtle particles from the food that it needs, and as the etheric body is the seat of vitality, memory and sensitivity, it is to your advantage to see that it is nourished.

The astral body is nourished by even more subtle matter than etheric particles: emotion, feelings. If you concentrate on the food you are eating with love, your astral body will extract from it the precious particles it needs and as a result, will be filled with love for the whole world... you will feel happy and at peace, with one desire only, to live in harmony with Nature. This sensation hardly exists today for humans no longer have that attitude of protectveness, of being careful and loving with objects, trees, mountains, stars, etc... they are too upset and worried about themselves and feel threatened even when they are safe at home or even asleep. Actually they are not threatened, the feeling of being abandoned by Mother Nature comes from the fact that their astral body has not been fed! When the astral body is properly nourished, you have a marvellous feeling of wellbeing that makes you want to behave generously and toler- antly in life, and if you have important problems to solve, you handle everything with tact and understanding, you know how to make conces- sions.

To nourish the mental body, the Initiate concentrates on his food with his eyes closed; as the food is for him a manifestation of God, he tries to see all its aspects, where it comes from, what it contains, what qualities it has, what enti- ties have cared for it... for there are invisible be- ings who take care of trees and plants. His mind is absorbed with these matters whilst he draws elements from the food that are still more subtle than those needed by the astral body. A meal partaken of in that way leaves him with a comprehension he did not have to start with, he sees all things more clearly and is ready to undertake the most exacting mental work.

Most people imagine it is through reading, studying and reflecting that one develops intellectual capacities... no, although study and reflection are certainly indispensable, in themselves they are not enough. The mental body needs to be fed certain elements during meals for it to be strong and resistant enough to make prolonged efforts.

You must understand that the astral body is what sustains your emotions, and the mental body sustains your mind, your thinking: these two bodies must therefore be given the appropriate nourishment before you can expect to be equal to the task of living your life.

Beyond the etheric, astral and mental bodies, man has other bodies made of a still more spiritual substance, the causal, buddhic and atmic bodies, or seat of reason, the soul, and the spirit, which must also be fed. Their nourishment is a feeling of gratitude toward God. Gratitude (which is also disappearing from human existence) is what opens the spiritual doors to all the blessings. Everything becomes clear, you see, you feel, you live! Gratitude transforms gross matter into light and joy. Learn to be thankful.

When you feed your three higher bodies, the subtle particles that you capture are distributed in the brain, the solar plexus and all the other organs. You realize that you have other higher needs, that joys of an infinitely superior nature exist for you, and this will open the door to greater possibilities.

Once you finish eating, you should not go back to arguing or working immediately, but neither should you stretch out on a chaise-longue for hours. By remaining quiet for an instant and breathing deeply, the energies you have acquired from the food will be distributed throughout the system and then you will be ready to undertake the most arduous work. Remember that the beginning is the most important moment in all activity!

2

HRANI-YOGA

At the present moment, people are unbalanced by the hectic life they lead and are willing to try anything in the hopes of regaining their equilibrium... yoga, Zen, transcendental meditation, 'relaxing'.... I have nothing against any of these things, but there is a simpler and more effective way of restoring balance, which is to learn to eat correctly.

When you eat carelessly and indifferently, in a rush, in the midst of noise, discussions, tension and pressure, what good is it to meditate or anything else afterwards? Play-acting! It would be better to use this opportunity you have two or three times a day, every day, to do something as you eat that will put all your cells in order and harmonize your entire system.

If I ask you to make an effort to eat in silence (refraining not only from talking, but also from making a noise with knives and forks, etc...) to chew each mouthful a long time and take a deep

breath from time to time, and above all, to thank
Heaven as you eat for all the riches the food contains... it is because these apparently insignificant exercises are the means of acquiring self-
control. By learning to control little things you
gain control over big things. When I see someone being negligent and careless in small matters, I know that his life has been disorderly in
the past and will be in the future unless he does
something about this failing. Because everything
is related.

I know it is not easy to remain silent during
meals and concentrate only on food, even if you
manage to be quiet and control your gestures,
inwardly you still make a noise with your feelings, or perhaps your feelings are under control
but your thoughts wander off. Nutrition is a
yoga in that when you are eating, you devote
your full efforts, your attention, concentration,
and control to the process of eating.

To be able to concentrate your thoughts during meals, you must have acquired the habit of
controlling your thoughts in daily life. If you
have always been careful not to let yourself be
invaded by negative thoughts and feelings, then,
yes, the way is paved and it will be easy for you.
You say, "Should an entire life be spent learning
to eat properly?" Yes, and no. All your problems are obviously not going to be solved simply

because you eat correctly, it is a point of departure, a springboard leading to extraordinarily beneficial things, but it doesn't mean that nothing else is important and that you can let yourself go the rest of the time! In short, it is desirable to eat your food attentively, with vigilance, and it is desirable to be attentive and vigilant during the rest of the day. One does not exclude the other.

Eating is a magic rite during which the food becomes transformed into health, force, love, light. Observe yourself, if you eat in a state of anger, agitation, discontent, you will be left with a bitter taste in your mouth all day, you will feel nervous and tense, and, if there are difficult problems to be solved, you will be negative in your reactions, your decisions will lack fairness and comprehension, you will not be generous enough to make concessions. It will do no good to justify yourself, "It isn't my fault, I am so nervous, I simply cannot help it!" and then swallow some medicine or other to try and calm yourself (which will do no good either). To improve your nervous system, you must learn to eat properly.

Everything else should be set aside when you sit down to eat, even important affairs, for the only important thing at that moment is to nourish yourself in compliance with divine rules. If

you eat correctly, the rest will take care of itself
when you have finished... in that way you save
both time and effort! You must not think it
solves problems better or more rapidly to be
tense and feverish about them, actually the re-
verse is true: you let things drop out of your
hands, you say things clumsily, you have a negative effect on others, after which you must spend
days making the necessary repairs.

Most humans cannot see that the smallest action in their daily lives is significant, so how can
they be expected to see that the way to develop
their intelligence, love and willpower, is to eat
properly? Everybody thinks of intelligence as
something you develop through reading and
studying, or through trials and tribulation when
you are forced to find a way out! They also
think the heart is awakened by having a wife and
children to take care of and protect, and that
willpower is something you develop through
physical effort, sport, etc... but to develop the
mind and heart and will during meals? Never!
Well, that kind of reasoning only proves that
they have not begun to understand the Teaching.

It is during meals that you do the real work,
the essential work, that is, develop your heart,
your mind and your will. Yes, it may be that you

are not able to spend all your time studying in libraries and universities, you may not get married and have children, you may not have the opportunity for prolonged and strenuous effort, but you will surely eat, everybody is obliged to eat!

Do you wish to develop your mind? Each time you handle something on the table during a meal, by doing it carefully without knocking things against each other, without disturbing anyone else, you develop your mind, you are becoming intelligent, attentive and perceptive. When I see people dropping their knives and forks, knocking things over, I know at once that they lack intelligence. They may have all kinds of degrees and diplomas, but for me they lack intelligence. What good is a degree if you are unable to gauge distances?

Let us say you wish to move a glass: unless you measure with your eye how far the glass is from other objects, you will knock something down and break it. This is a detail, a small failing, you say, but a failing that may well be blown up to giant proportions by coming events in your life. People who are awkward and careless during meals are awkward and careless in life (and cause great damage). To be inattentive on either a small scale or a large one, to blunder, wound people, upset things carelessly are all part of an attitude that causes suffering and resentment that may take years to repair.

Before I pick up this bottle of water on the table before me, I remind myself that it has been in the refrigerator, it may be damp and slippery and, if I am not careful in handling it, it may slip out of my hands and drop. To prevent that, I wipe it off before grasping it, and then I am sure it will not fall. That is the way it must be for everything, on the dinner table or in life. If something is outside your range of consciousness it will be outside your control, you will not be its master and it will not obey you. To control something you must dominate it in thought.

Another thing, before sitting down to dinner, try to make sure nothing is lacking so as not to have to get up again to fetch the salt, a plate, a knife. Often when I am invited, the hostess has to leave the table several times because she has forgotten something, yet she ought to know what is needed, she repeats the same identical thing each day! But no one pays attention and so a whole life is spent interrupting meals to fetch something you forgot. It is a sure sign that you are no more attentive and careful in bigger matters: will that lead to success?

If you try to eat without making a noise or

disturbing the others around you who need quiet in order to concentrate and meditate, it will develop your heart. People think, "The others? What are the others to me?" and that is why the whole world is degenerating, no one thinks about the others. Humans are not able to live with each other because they have no respect, no thoughtfulness for each other. Eating together offers them a chance to develop their character and enlarge their consciousness.

This is why I say that during meals you can learn control by surveying your gestures and refraining from making a noise. I know I am asking you something extremely hard to realize but if you can manage it, everyone who comes here will be astounded, they will say, "But it isn't possible, I don't believe my eyes!" My answer will be, "Well, then, believe your ears!"

You can tell how far along in his evolution a person is by whether or not he is conscious of belonging not only to himself, but to a whole, and the harmony of that whole must not be disturbed by his actions, thoughts or feelings, his inner noise. You say, "What does that mean, his inner noise?" Noise is dissonance, we make a noise inside ourselves with our pain and anguish, our rebelliousness and discontent, and it disturbs the psychic atmosphere of the whole.

We don't realize how bad this noise is for ourselves and for everyone else until the day comes when our system breaks down and there is psychic or physical illness to face.

Whilst you eat you should think of the food with love, for that will make it open its treasures to you... when the sun warms the flowers, they open up; when it disappears, they close. If you love food, if you eat it lovingly, it will open and exhale a fragrance for you and give you the etheric particles you are looking for. You will see what a marvellous state you will be in once you stop eating automatically with no love, simply to fill the void in your stomach.

I know it is useless to speak this way about love; humans do not know how to treat each other with love, how to talk, walk, look and breathe with love, how to greet each other and work with love... they don't know how! They think love consists in going to bed with someone, but the results prove that is not love : if they really knew how to love each other, Heaven would be there with them.

During meals you can develop your mind and your heart and also your will, since to acquire the habit of making restrained, deliberate, harmonious gestures, you are using willpower! When you feel nervous, seize the next mealtime as the opportunity to calm yourself, chew very slowly and be careful of every gesture : in a few minutes you will be calm again and at peace. If you start the day in a state of agitation and go to work or talk with someone without doing something to change the way you feel, you will remain agitated all day and your energy will evaporate : you forgot to close the tap! There is a simple and effective remedy for nerves, which is to stop everything and remain without talking for a second or two whilst you make a conscious effort to change your rhythm, choose another direction, and then start out again.

When you eat in silence and inner peace, the same peaceful state lasts all day, even if you have to run hither and thither all day, if you stop for a second you will see that the peace is still there. Because you ate correctly. If not, you will be agitated and upset, nervous and tense, all day long, no matter what you try to do to calm yourself.

The day is coming when nutrition will be considered the best of all yogas in spite of not having been mentioned before now. All the others, Radja-Yoga, Karma-Yoga, Hatha-Yoga, Jnani-Yoga, Agni-Yoga, are wonderful, but it takes years to obtain the slightest result, whereas with Hrani-Yoga as I call it (Hrani means food in Bulgarian), the results are immediate. It is the easiest yoga to learn, all creatures practise it unconsciously! This yoga so little known, so widely misunderstood, has everything, all the alchemy, all the magic.

Even if you are snowed under with work or things to do, do not try to hide behind the pretext of having no time for the spiritual life... three times a day, every day (since everyone eats three times a day), you have the best conditions you could have for communicating with Heaven, with God. You may have no time for prayer, for reading or meditating, granted, but everyone takes the time to eat! Why not use this moment to go a step further toward perfection by sending God a thought full of love and gratitude?

Begin today to make your meals a time for spiritual work, the work that is so necessary, so indispensable. People think they are already perfect (why not, they conform to the laws of society, they harm no one, they fulfill their professional and family duties...) but unless they do the spiritual work the divine world will remain closed to them and they will never taste the joy, happiness, plenitude and fulfilment, the Light that the divine life brings. They are perfect, yes, but what is this strange perfection that has no time for the soul and spirit?

Of course, everyone has to work for a living,

in order to survive without being a burden to others, but everyone must also take at least a few minutes to nourish the soul and spirit. We have all come on this earth with a mission, but most people are too busy thinking of their social success, believing they are perfect... why is it that no light emanates from them if they are perfect? Because they have no time, either for the spiritual life or for their own improvement.

We are here on earth for a very short time, and when we leave we will not be able to take any of our material acquisitions with us, no cars, no houses, no possessions... all that will be left behind, we will only be allowed our inner acquisitions. That is what you have never really understood, and it is why you are always immersed in material activities. What for? You will have to abandon everything when you go, you will be naked, poor and miserable.

Now you know that you should work spiritually during meals! The results may not show at once, maybe no one will appreciate what you are trying to do, but go ahead, keep on storing up spiritual riches by developing the best qualities and virtues within yourself. When you come back in your next incarnation, Heaven will give you better conditions to help you blossom forth, because of the fact that you have begun the work, the real work, in this incarnation. This truth taken from the divine Science is for you, you should know it, and even if you do not accept it, eventually it will triumph, eventually it will enlighten you and you will be saved.

3

A LETTER FROM GOD

Take a fruit... without for the moment going into its taste, perfume or colour, let us concentrate on the idea that it is a letter written by our Creator with rays of sun, and that our life depends on the way we read this letter. If we do not know how to read, we will not draw much benefit from it... what a pity!

A girl or boy who receives a letter from the one they love, see how fervently they read and reread it, how carefully they handle it, how precious it is to them. We toss the love letter we receive from God into the wastebasket... does it not merit reading? Man is the only creature who makes no effort to decipher this letter, even animals are more interested... yes, cattle for instance, they know when they have not read it properly and read it over again! You are laughing at this unscientific explanation... very well, call it ruminating to be scientific, but I say, they are rereading their letter from God.

Fruit is a love letter from God that needs to be deciphered. It is the most eloquent, the most stirring of love letters, since it says, "You are loved! Someone cares for you so much that He wants you to have life, and is sending you the means to live!" Humans prefer to swallow in a hurry and make no attempt to read what He says, "My child, I want you to become like this fruit, tasty and sweet and perfect. Right now you are hard and sour, still unripe, and so you must learn. This fruit became ripe by being exposed to the sun: be like the fruit, expose yourself to the sun, the spiritual sun, and it will transform you from something acid and indigestible into a being with heavenly colours." That is what God has put in the food for us to hear and act upon, you may not hear Him, but I do.

If we know how to listen, food speaks to us. Food is condensed light and sound, but if your thoughts are busy elsewhere, you cannot hear the 'voice' of the light. Light and sound are not separate things, light sings, light is music. You should listen to the music of light: it is the sacred Word.

One might also say that food is a kind of radiesthesia. Each being, each object, has its own particular radiation, and a radiesthesist is one who grasps these radiations and interprets them. The food we eat has received radiations from everywhere in the cosmos, the sun, the stars, the four elements, and all these radiations have left imprints that are invisible but nonetheless real, in the form of forces and particles of energy. It has recorded traces of all the beings who walked and worked in the fields where it grew and it will tell you (if you can hear) the stories of how God, the sun, the stars, the angels and humans worked on it night and day, filling it with properties that are helpful to men, God's children.

Although Nature sees how ignorant and somnolent humans are, she is so generous that she says, "Bah, no matter! I will fill their food with the forces that keep them alive whether they are conscious or not." When man is as unconscious in his eating as animals are, the food helps them to grow physically, it keeps them alive, but it will not help them spiritually.

To receive the most subtle particles in the food, you must be fully conscious, wide awake, full of love. If the entire system is ready to receive food in that perfect way, then the food is moved to pour out its hidden riches. Like someone you receive with love, he opens himself and gives you everything he has; if you are cold, he remains closed. Expose a flower to warmth and light, it will open and give you its perfume, but if you leave it in the dark, out in the cold, it will not open. Food also remains open or closed depending upon the attitude of the one who partakes of it : when food opens itself, it gives you all that it has in the way of pure, divine energies.

4

CHOOSING YOUR FOOD

I

One day, one of the sisters who is a doctor received a telephone call from a lady whose husband was laid low with a liver attack. "Could it be something he ate?" asked the lady. "Yesterday we went to a wedding reception...." "Ah," said our sister. "What did you eat?" "Not much as far as I was concerned," was the answer. "I was not hungry, but my husband has a very good appetite and he ate what was offered..." and she described the menu. It was unbelievable! Ham and sausages and pâté and melon, sweetbread with clams, trout with almonds, rabbit with prunes, cake with cream, cheeses, puddings, fruit, wine, Champagne, coffee, liqueurs.... "Do you think there might have been something in the food that made him ill?" she ended. As you can see, some people see no connection between what they consume in the way of food and the state of their health.

Nevertheless, man builds his body with the

food he absorbs, it is formed by what he consumes and for that reason you should stop thinking that you will be beaming with health no matter what you swallow, you must realize that a rapport exists between what you eat and the way you feel. When you fill yourself with incongruous mixtures, your system will not be able to eliminate them and you will fall ill. It is important to be careful what you take into your body.

Someone will bring up the verse in the Gospels in which Jesus says that it is not what enters into a man but what comes out of him, that is important... but that too must be interpreted. Is it rational to think that if you put filth into something it will be purity that comes out? Unless you are an Initiate with the ability to transform whatever you eat into light. Yes, but that takes an Initiate! The others, if they take in filth, it will be filth that comes out. They cannot possibly transform anything if they are neither intelligent nor pure, neither loving nor kind.

Jesus never gave the advice to eat or drink anything regardless, nor would an Initiate do so. Only if you know how to work spiritually and can neutralize poison and impurity and transform them into light are you free to swallow anything you wish. And the opposite, if you have not yet decided to work spiritually, the best food in the world will not be able to transform you. It is the powerful inner life of thought and feeling that is essential.

I know that diet experts favour certain foods over others... and they may be right... but first and foremost it is the way you eat that is important. Eat what you like, but only if you eat it in a certain way and in reasonable quantities will you be healthy. The quantities of people who go on macrobiotic or other diets do not become better or stronger I have noticed, but rather the contrary, they are feebler and worse off than before. I have nothing against macrobiotics or anything else, I recognize that there may be some good in those things, but I do not agree that food or eating should be put in first place as the most important thing in life. Food is only a means, the important thing is the psychic life, the spiritual life behind the action of eating.

No amount of wonderful food has ever kept anyone from being cruel or wicked or depraved, or from wanting to dominate the world. To be a vegetarian is no help apparently: Hitler was a vegetarian! Whilst others who became saints and prophets, ate meat or anything else they were given. With no schooling, no hygiene, no food except what came their way, but with what they considered the most important, the spirit, a few truths, and the indomitable will to realize these truths, they worked miracles!

Let us come back to the food we eat every day. On the physical plane our food will never be absolutely pure of course, most of the time you do not know what you are given, but in the realm of thoughts and feelings it is different, you can choose what you like, allowing yourself only the best and discarding the rest. Thoughts and feelings are the substance our subtler bodies are made of, and if we build a hovel, symbolically speaking, then it will not be a Prince or a High Priest who will visit us, but a beggar or a thief. We build our etheric, astral and mental bodies ourself, and our destiny depends on the materials we use. According to the quality of our subtler bodies we will be visited by shining entities or dark ones, blessed with joy or suffering, achieve true glory or end up in darkness.

The future of each one of us depends on the way we nourish ourselves. When you eat inferior food on the physical plane, what happens? It shows in the way you look and feel and people ask you what is wrong. If the quality of the food you eat changes your appearance, why wouldn't it be the same for the quality of your thoughts and feelings? Some thoughts, some feelings, make you beautiful and healthy and others make you ugly and sickly... why not take this into consideration and act accordingly?

Before transforming himself, man must have

acquired new particles of a better, finer quality. Merely to observe silence during meals is not enough therefore, we must fill this silence with our most elevated thoughts and feelings if it is to have the powerful, magical element that is the proper nourishment for our subtler bodies. Silence should not be a void, in Nature there is no such thing, every space is filled with forces and elements that become purer and purer the higher they are, and the closer to heavenly regions. Silence is a magic goldmine full of riches to be drawn upon.

II

The four elements (earth, water, air, fire) correspond with the four states of matter contained in the food we absorb each day. We should communicate with the Angels of these elements as we eat, the Angel of Earth, the Angel of Water, the Angel of Air, the Angel of Fire, and ask them to rebuild our physical body and make it so pure that it will be fit for the Christ, the Living God to come and dwell in.

Each Angel represents a determined virtue or quality: the Angel of Earth, stability; the Angel of Water, purity; the Angel of Air, intelligence; the Angel of Fire, Divine Love. If, while eating, man links himself in thought to these four Angels, the particles he receives will be spiritual ones with which he can build his subtle bodies... including the body of light. When he is able to build that luminous body called in the Scriptures the Body of Glory, then he is truly immortal. His physical body does not last long, he must give it back with all its elements to the mother earth whence it came. But in his body of light, the Body of Glory, man lives eternally.

The Body of Glory is an etheric seed, a tiny seed or electron which we inherit and which must be developed, fed and formed by ourselves, in the same way that a mother works for months on the seed she receives from the father, adding the best material she can in order to form a living being able to stir up the world, so we must work on the spiritual plane to form and feed and develop our Body of Glory. If we never think about it, if we do nothing, then it remains hidden, cast aside, buried. Fortunately it does not die for it is deathless, but it waits in its hidden state until our consciousness awakens and we do the work that will develop it and make it luminous and powerful.

Intensely pure elements are needed to develop the Body of Glory, only the most intense vibrations of light can fight against the process of illness and death, disorganization, fermentation, disintegration, but when the light triumphs in a man, he is immortal. For that reason, you must learn how to eat and drink the light as you eat, having the absolute certainty that your food is bringing you the new life.

If you communicate with the Angels of the

four elements as you eat, they will become your friends and collaborators. Forget all your little worries and grudges, your wicked thoughts that poison the food and make you ill, and link yourself with the Angels of the four elements. Say, "O Angel of the Earth, fill me with your stability! O Angel of Water, fill me with your purity! O Angel of Air, fill me with your intelligence! O Angel of Fire, fill me with your Divine Love!" In this manner you will be born into the new life.

5

VEGETARIANISM

The question of nutrition is a far-reaching one that has many ramifications. We are nourished not only by the food and drink we consume during meals, but by other things as well, such as sounds, colours, odours. The idea that in the invisible world there are beings who nourish themselves on fragrant (or evil) smells, gave rise to the tradition of burning incense in churches, for pure and fragrant odours attract shining spirits, and nauseous odours attract diabolical entities. Spirits also feed on sound and colour, and these can be used as a means to attract them. The great painters knew this, they depicted Angels in shining colours, playing heavenly music on their golden instruments.

It says in the Gospels, "Ye are the temple of the living God." If this is our belief, why do we soil this temple with impurities? If humans realized how they were created in the first place, in the Lord's workshops, they would be more careful about the material they use to construct this temple in which God may come and dwell. The fact that man eats meat makes him more like a cemetery full of rotting corpses than a temple.

Every creature, animal or human, is free to choose his nutrition, and this choice is highly significant. If you want to know the effects of a carnivorous diet, go and visit the zoo, look at the carnivores and you will know all you need to know about the effects of eating meat! Actually it is not even necessary to go so far, human beings reflect every known specimen of animal, and even some that are not known, nor found in zoos, such as dinosaurs, mammoths and other prehistoric monsters! But let us be charitable and confine ourselves to the zoo: you will verify for yourselves that the big carnivorous mammals are fearful beasts that exude extremely strong odours, whilst the herbivores have peaceful habits because their food does not make them violent and aggressive. Carnivores are rendered irritable and violent by their diet of meat and it is the same for humans: those who eat meat are more brutal and destructive than vegetarians.

The difference between vegetarian and carnivorous food lies in the amount of solar rays they contain: fruit and vegetables are impregnated with solar light to such an extent that you might say they are condensed light. By eating fruit or vegetables, you absorb solar light and there is practically no waste matter involved. Meat on the other hand, is comparatively poor in solar light and for that reason, spoils rapidly... anything that spoils rapidly is bad for the health.

Still another danger exists from eating meat. When animals are being led to the slaughter-house, they sense what lies ahead and it terrifies them, they are literally panic-stricken. This fear fills the glands with a lethal secretion that permeates the system of whoever eats their flesh... with disastrous effects on his health and life-span. You say, "Yes, but meat is so delicious!" There you go again, thinking only of your personal gratification! All that interests you is your pleasure, all that counts is the moment, even though it means that millions of animals will be massacred... and yourself as well.

You should know that everything you absorb in the way of food becomes a sort of inner antenna that captures different waves... meat links you with the lower regions of the astral world and the beings who devour each other like wild beasts. The meat is an invisible link to brute fear, cruelty, sensuality: the animal world. Anyone who is able to see colours would be distressed at the colours in your aura.

Lastly, it is a grave responsibility to take the life of an animal. Not only is it transgressing the law, "Thou shalt not kill," but it is robbing the animal of the chance to evolve during its present existence. To kill an animal is to take not only its life, but the chance Nature has given it to evolve. The animal soul is not the same as the human soul, but it is still a soul, and the person who eats meat carries animal souls around with him, manifesting through him in bestial ways. In the invisible world the souls of the animals killed and eaten by a man attach themselves to him and ask to be compensated, "You deprived us of the opportunity to evolve and now it is up to you to give us the education of which you robbed us." This explains why so many humans have animal reactions, and if they ever try to develop their higher nature, they will be prevented from doing so by the animal cells within that refuse to obey.

In Genesis, it says that before the Fall when God was creating man's physical sustenance, He said simply, "Behold, I have given you every herb-bearing seed which is upon the face of all the earth and every tree in which is the fruit of a tree yielding seed, to you it shall be for meat."

Concerning fish, the problem is different. For

millions of years fish have existed without proper conditions for evolution, they have a very rudimentary nervous system, so that one might say to eat them makes them evolve... besides the fact that fish contain an element called iodine, which was designed for this epoch.

The food we eat goes into our bloodstream and from there attracts entities that correspond to it in nature. The Gospel says, "Wheresoever the carcass is there the eagles will be gathered together," and this truth applies on all planes, the physical, astral and mental. If you wish to be healthy, do not attract eagles (or vultures) with carcasses on any plane! Heaven will not manifest through anyone who is open to physical, astral or mental impurity.

Meat corresponds to a certain element in our thoughts, feelings and actions. For instance, if you dream that you are eating meat, you should be extremely careful, for it means you are facing temptation of a certain kind, leading to acts of violence, sensual feelings, or egotistical, unjust thoughts: meat represents violence on the physical plane, sensuality on the astral plane, and egoism on the mental plane.

Tradition says that before the Fall, Adam had a beautiful shining face and was beloved of animals, all of which respected and obeyed him.

After the Fall, Adam lost this pure and shining visage and the animals became his enemies. Beasts do not trust man, birds fly away at his approach, all Creation thinks of him as an enemy, and there must be a reason : it is because he has fallen from the spiritual heights. Now he can regain his original splendour by submitting to the laws of love and wisdom as he once did, and becoming reconciled to all Creation. When he does, it will bring the Kingdom of God on earth.

Wars are in appearance brought about by problems of economics, politics, etc... but actually they are the result of the way humans slaughter animals. The law of justice is implacable. Man must pay with his blood for all the blood he has spilt, human or animal. Millions of litres of blood crying vengeance to Heaven have soaked into this earth, its evaporation attracts not only microbes but billions of larvae and lower entities from the invisible world. These truths are still unknown to you, and to most people and will probably not be accepted, but I am obliged to reveal them whether you accept them or not.

And so we go on killing animals. We do not realize that Nature is one vast organism, a system whose functioning is disturbed by the murder of so many of its cells, it creates an imbalance, and we should not be surprised when wars break out. Yes, millions of animals are slaughtered by us for human consumption, without our knowing that in the invisible world these animals are linked to humans, and it is therefore humans that we kill: by killing animals, we kill men. Everyone talks about outlawing war and bringing peace to the world at all costs, but peace cannot exist on earth as long as we go on killing animals, because when we kill them, we are killing ourselves.

6

THE MORAL ASPECT

People imagine they should eat great quantities of food in order to be strong and healthy, but actually, you tire the system when you overload it, the digestive process is impeded, and when the system is not able to eliminate properly, then illness appears... all because of the erroneous idea that you must eat a lot in order to be healthy.

In actual fact, a little hunger prolongs life! If you always eat to your fill and are stuffed after every meal, you lack energy, you are heavy and somnolent and do not feel like doing the work of perfecting yourself. If, on the other hand, you leave the table still slightly hungry, refusing a few mouthfuls you would have liked, the etheric body, in order to compensate, goes looking in the higher regions for the elements you need. Instead of being hungry you feel alive and light and ready to work, because the etheric body has absorbed elements that are superior to ordinary

food. Eating your fill or more, if you are one of
those who enjoy eating to excess, throws your
system out of balance, and you will never have
enough.

Besides weighing down the system when you
eat too much, you also prevent your etheric
body from functioning as it should... which
opens the door to entities from the lower astral
plane: seeing the abundance of food you have
unconsciously offered them, they rush to the
feast! A few minutes later you feel hungry all
over again. The void is there perpetually, always
demanding more, and each time the undesirables come back. You yourself are keeping all
the thieving, starving undesirables on the lower
astral plane well-nourished... at your expense.

When I say to leave the table still feeling
hungry, I mean only very slightly hungry, for if
you deny your system everything, the etheric
body cannot make up the difference. But if you
forego say twenty grams or so out of every kilo,
then because of the etheric element that is added, you will feel light and eager to work. How
many times have I verified this! You say, "But it
is such a temptation to take more!" I know, but
what about willpower, what about your deci-
sion... this is the moment to try it out! At din-
ner-parties and receptions also you must learn to
refuse, as I do. Whenever I am invited to dinner,

even though I tell my hosts in advance not to make a fuss, not to prepare anything special but to give me a little salad, vegetable and fruit, no more... no one pays any attention, they always prepare a sumptuous repast and when they see how little I eat, they are disappointed! They should listen to what I say!

I understood long ago that by eating too much one loses something more precious and subtle than physical food has to offer, no matter how succulent the dish. You must learn to refuse when you are offered too much, otherwise you will be too full, too soggy and sleepy to do anything worthwhile, the spiritual work is put aside, and there it waits. Do not sleep, there is work to do!

Of course, it is up to each one to know how much food to eat, not everyone has the same capacity. I have seen some phenomenal eaters in my life, like Tseko for instance, a brother of the Fraternity in Bulgaria. He had the most astounding appetite, he never had enough! He was the nicest, most willing fellow, always smiling, good-natured and because he was tremendously strong, he was made to carry all the baggage when we went to camp on top of Moussala. They (the older sisters especially) would load him down like a donkey, but he accepted without a murmur. Looking back at him on the way, he looked like a whole mountain of luggage advancing along the path! Sometimes the brothers and sisters would load the samovar on his back in order to make tea once at the top, a whole samovar complete with glowing cinders. If the water started to boil as it sometimes did, you would hear the kettle whistling whilst Tseko advanced steadily like a locomotive, with the steam pouring out of the samovar!

His good nature made him enormously popular and he was invited everywhere, but wherever he went, he ate everything in sight. If something was left over, it had to be removed at once from the table or Tseko would devour it, it would disappear into his enormous stomach! When we broke camp at Rila, we usually carried the food that had gone bad back down with us, but when the sisters who did the cooking went to get it, it would have vanished... Tseko again! But he was never ill. The Master Peter Deunov knew about his phenomenal appetite, and whenever there was someone with us who had lost his appetite, he would seat him next to Tseko: inevitably, watching him eat, his appetite would return! What a phenomenon!

That was not all there was to Tseko. Virtually illiterate, almost completely uneducated, he began one day to write poetry. To him poetry was a simple question of rhymes; his verses did indeed rhyme, but they made no sense! When he read his poems aloud, everyone laughed, it was impossible not to, but although he knew we were poking fun at him, he remained imperturbable, unruffled, never upset, always smiling and ready to read his poetry to us as we sat before the fire under the stars at Rila. One day his rhymes turned into real poetry and we stopped laughing. Then he decided to compose music and wrote some songs. At first we made fun of him, Tesko the composer! But soon you could hear the brothers and sisters all over the mountain singing Tseko's compositions as they walked around the lakes.

He was an electrician by profession, and one day to our grief we learned that the current had passed through him as he worked on an electric pole and he had fallen to his death. That is how he died. Everyone grieved. Even now, fifty years or so later, I often think about him. In any case, I never again saw such a stomach!

But you are not Tseko, and you should know that too much food is bad for your health. Besides, when you eat more than is necessary for your proper sustenance, you are taking away from others, and if everyone did that, it would throw the world out of balance. Misunderstandings, revolutions, wars, have one thing at their origin : greed, the cupidity of people who can afford to accumulate all kinds of things, food, ·land, objects, to the deprivation of others. The collective consciousness is not yet sufficiently awakened to realize this, nor to foresee the consequences of inordinate greed.

The need to take and absorb more than one needs, more than one's share, is also what makes people want to subjugate and dominate, even kill, others. Insignificant and minute as it may seem, this is the starting point for all catastrophes. We must be taught from our youngest age to control, to measure and regulate this instinct ; if not, it will assume giant proportions in every realm of our existence and be for us a source of great unhappiness.

That is the reason a disciple should learn not to go beyond certain limits when he eats, to stop before he has had his fill. By not knowing when to stop, he feeds his unnatural desires and becomes like people who have too much money and want to own everything... they already have everything they need, but their ambition and greed are such that they want to swallow the entire world.

Jesus said that it is easier for a camel to pass through the eye of a needle than for a rich man to enter the Kingdom of God. For 2 000 years this image has remained unexplained and if you

cannot see the hidden meaning it is a strange
image indeed. Actually, Jesus was referring not
to the physical body, but to the astral body: the
astral body of a rich man, the body of desire,
when it is distended by excessive greed, becomes
a tumour, an immense tumour that prevents
him from being able to pass through the gates of
the Kingdom of God, wide as they are. The astral body of a camel on the other hand, is small,
his desires are few, he is content with very little.
That is what enables him to cross the desert, to
keep going when everyone else has given up.

And so, you see, that is what happens: those
who do not think this way, who eat too much on
every plane, develop tumours in their astral bodies that prevent them from going through the
doors leading to Initiation. They are also incur-
ring debts by taking what belongs to others, an
attitude that goes against the law of the spiritual
world which demands an organized, harmonious, just and equitable distribution of things.

If the Higher Beings see that your mentality
is selfish and coarse, they will not accept you
amongst them, they will say, "Stay there in the
jungle with the beasts devouring each other...
that is where you belong." Even if you complain
that you are being devoured and stung, nothing
will help, you will have to suffer. Until you
adopt the philosophy of the Great Universal

White Brotherhood the doors of Heaven will be closed to you.

You must understand that nutrition is not only a question of physical nourishment, the same laws exist in the realm of thoughts and feelings. Lovers who eat to the point of satiety form tumours in their astral bodies that will close the doors of Heaven to them. The proof that Heaven is not with them is that they are soon disgusted, their inspiration leaves them, they separate or even kill each other.

Now drop this idea that you must eat a lot of food in order to be healthy. A mother will think she is doing her child a favour (she loves him so much) by stuffing him with food. Stupid mother! Instead she should teach him to measure things carefully, to understand that by taking more for himself than he actually needs (of whatever it may be), he is depriving someone else, if not on the physical plane, then on the astral or mental planes. We must think about others! How many of us ever divide our wealth once we gain it, I mean the wealth of our thoughts and feelings? When you are in a wondrous state, when you feel rich and happy over something that causes you joy and wonderment, do you think of distributing that wealth to those near you who are in misery, or do you keep it all? When you overflow with happiness, give a little of this abundance, say, "Dear brothers and sisters of the world, what I have is so abundant and wonderful that I want to share it with you: take some of this happiness, take some of this joy, take some of this light!" If you can do that, if your consciousness is developed enough for you to feel that way, then your name will be inscribed in the heavenly records as beings intelligent and loving. What you distribute will be credited to your account for you to draw upon when you need to, and your joy will remain intact, no one can take it from you because you have put it in a safe place.

Furthermore, if you will observe yourself, you will see that when you hold on to a joy without sharing it, something happens to it, the malevolent beings in the invisible world (who are constantly watching) take it away from you through someone or something close to you. You lose your joy because you did not think of giving it to God, to the Divine Mother, saying, "O Lord, O Divine Mother, I am too stupid to know how to distribute this joy and so I give it to you to distribute as you see fit." They will see it and make a deposit in the heavenly banks. In that way, not only will you be helped, but you are benefiting the whole world.

From now on remember to keep within reasonable limits as far as food is concerned and remember also that when you eat, it is not only a question of physical food. Besides, if you learn to eat consciously and with love, even if you cut down on the amount, you will be drawing an incredible amount of energy. A single mouthful eaten that way gives sufficient energy to send a train around the world... yes, one mouthful!

7

FASTING

I

Fasting as Purification

You know that when you eat, your system absorbs what it needs and tries to get rid of what is foreign or harmful to it. The system is not able to do this eliminating when it has been over-charged or when the food it is given contains too many impurities. The waste matter then accumulates in the different organs, especially in the intestines.

How can you distinguish pure food from impure food? Food that putrifies rapidly and leaves a lot of waste matter in the system is not pure, even when washed and cooked, it is still impure. Food that does not decay rapidly, such as fruit which keeps fresh for a long time, and vegetables that are full of solar energy, is pure.

Even when it is pure, food leaves behind a lot of waste matter in the system, which is why the Initiates advise fasting from time to time to rid the physical body of impurities. Fasting is advocated by Nature... animals know instinctively that they must fast and eat grass to purge themselves when they are sick. When your furniture is covered with dust, you wipe it off, but when it is a question of cleaning your own organism at least once a week so that the millions of workers, the cells of your body, will be able to rest... you do nothing. Sometimes you have a fever, a runny nose and eyes, eruptions on your skin: it is a purification. Humans are too stubborn to purify themselves and the organs are compelled to do it for them.

I advise fasting twenty-four hours each week: for twenty-four hours take nothing but hot boiled water, nothing else. During that time you work spiritually, thinking about the higher beings, listening to good music and reading inspiring books, to purify your thoughts and feelings as well as the physical body. If you do that regularly you will ascertain that the waste matter you eliminate has no odor... do not be shocked, think of me for the moment as a doctor: if the waste matter discharged by your intestines and perspiration has a strong unpleasant odour, you can be sure that you are either ill or going to be, physically or psychically. You reply that odours depend on the food you take in... no, if you watch yourself carefully you will see that when you have been anxious and overwrought, angry or jealous, the odour changes. One's odour is very revealing.

I receive many letters (especially from women) saying, "I am willing to fast, but when I do, I become ugly!" Yes, perhaps in the beginning, but that only proves the presence of a lot of refuse that must be got rid of. At the start you may also have headaches, palpitations, fainting spells, but there is nothing to be afraid of, it is natural. No one has ever died from fasting occasionally, but thousands and thousands die from overeating! It may be new and upsetting for the system to begin with, but it is only momentary and in fact a good sign. If you can stand a little discomfort and keep on with your fast, you will see that in a day or two the inner disorder gives way to an extraordinary tranquility.

You must not judge fasting by the first effects, there is no danger involved, on the contrary, people who are disturbed are the very ones who need to fast most, the disturbance is caused by the superabundant waste matter being discharged into the bloodstream by the cleansing. People think that fasting weakens them and gives them an unhealthy look, which could be true at the beginning but when you become lighter, your skin clears up and you are more pleasant to look at! If you don't know the language of Nature, you can be scared to death by a little discomfort. You think, "With these palpitations, I may die, I feel weak!" and start eating again, congesting your system just as it was beginning to emerge from all the encumbrance. As the disturbances cease when you resume eating, you conclude that you were right in interrupting the fast, but it is not so.

People who are seriously interested in fasting must learn to think differently. If they feel upset they must pay no attention but keep on until the disturbances stop, which will be shortly. The disturbances are the result of Nature trying to rid the organism of waste matter, and the best thing is to wait until that is done. By refusing to wait, you make the same mistake as people who take pills to stop a fever. It may make them feel better for the moment, but to bring a fever down that way paves the way for a much more serious illness. It is better to let the system react by itself. When the system is overcharged, it reacts by doing everything it can to eliminate waste matter, and this process of dissolving or eliminating the waste is what gives you a temperature, it is the inner cleansing that causes it. How can you help the system do this cleansing? By drinking water, boiling hot water. Several cups in succession will bring the fever down immediately: the canals dilate and the blood circulates freely, bearing the waste matter out of the body through the normal channels....

Hot water is essential when you are fasting. Bring it to a boil to kill the germs, and let it settle. When you wash dishes in cold water, the plates are still greasy; hot water is also needed to dissolve grease in the organism, it dissolves substances that cold water leaves intact, and draws them out of the body through the pores and kidneys, etc... and you are rejuvenated! You might drink hot water every day before breakfast, it is an excellent remedy against arteriosclerosis, rheumatism, etc....

Hot water may not be appetizing at first, but little by little you will begin to feel so well that it becomes a pleasure. Hot water is an extraordinary remedy, but it is so simple, so cheap, that no one takes it seriously. One of the brothers cured himself that way of an illness that his doctor had been unable to cure. When the brother went back to the doctor, cured, the latter said, "Yes, I know hot water works miracles in many cases, but how can I charge a consultation fee for prescribing hot water?"

When you fast, your etheric body goes to work to bring the physical body purer, more subtle elements, it watches over the physical body and restores its energy when needed; fasting makes the etheric body work, during which time the physical body rests. If the fast lasts too long, the etheric body is overworked, it has more than it can handle alone. The physical body and the etheric body are partners and if only one does the work, the balance is disturbed.

I have told you that one of the most important rules of nutrition is to stop eating *before* you are full. Why? Because if you get up from the table still hungry, your system reacts to this insufficiency and the etheric body supplies what is lacking... that is why if you wait a little, you are no longer hungry and you feel much better than if you had eaten your fill. Always leave the table slightly hungry. People think it is better to eat a lot, but nothing makes you grow old faster than loading the stomach.

When I say to leave the table hungry, I mean a very slight hunger. If you deprive the system of something it needs over a long period of time, the etheric body is not able to take care of it, but if you eat a little less than you are used to, you will feel lighter and better disposed toward life because of the added etheric element. If you eat too much you will feel heavy and sleepy. Why? Because sleep is necessary while the etheric body rids the system of the burdensome food. If the surplus must be removed, why add it in the first place?

You think that what I am saying is not very important and is certainly not an Initiatic subject, but if you leave the table each time feeling slightly empty, if you fast and drink hot water from time to time, you will see tremendous benefits even in your spiritual life.

I will add a few words on the way you should end a fast that has lasted several days... if you eat normally at once it can be fatal. The first day, take a few cups of bouillon; the next day, soup and biscuits; the third day begin to eat normally again, but not too much. In that way you risk nothing; after such a fast you are filled with new, subtle and wonderful feelings and revelations, you feel and look younger, freer, as if something heavy in your system has been burned away with the impurities. It is fear and ignorance that have kept humans from fasting and being regenerated.

II

Fasting as a Form of Nourishment

The question of fasting is more far-reaching than it appears to be. Man attracts the misfortunes that befall him because of the impurity within him left over from his past lives. Every sin, every fault and error, has left its mark, the dregs are still there, inside. By fasting you get rid of these impurities, and the light can shine through, making you feel lighter and happier! For that reason the great spiritual teachers of all religions have always prescribed fasting.

To fast does not mean to deprive yourself, on the contrary, fasting is less a form of renouncement than of nourishment. When the physical body is deprived of food, the other bodies (etheric, astral, mental) have to do the work. There is a principle in every man compelling him to make every effort to keep from dying, and when the physical body is not fed properly, the alert goes out to the entities in the higher regions to come to the rescue with finer elements culled from the atmosphere. If the person who is fasting interrupts his breathing at that moment for a second, entities from still higher regions will come bearing the very highest form of nourishment.

The Initiates tell us that the first man nourished himself with fire and light. In the course of man's involution he descended further and further into matter and his needs became progressively heavier and denser until he was obliged to nourish himself as he does now. That is why the Initiates, realizing that the way we eat now is the result of involution, make every attempt to return to the original state of man, by learning how to capture and absorb the subtlest and finest elements. They control their intake, as if they temporarily rejected first their stomach and then their lungs, in order to liberate their thoughts. This requires long and arduous discipline, even in India very few yogis have control over their respiration. Those who have this control can swim in the Akasha, the cosmic ether, and acquire total knowledge for they are totally free.

Man descended from the celestial regions by the process of involution. As he descended into matter and entered the cold regions at the periphery, his body grew heavier and denser until it became the physical body as we know it. We

do the same thing in winter when we put on our
heavier clothes to protect us from the cold.
Now, before man can take the upward path, before he can go back up to the heights, he must,
symbolically speaking, get rid of everything that
weighs him down. Fasting is the means of becoming light again, of recovering his original
lightness and purity.

The point of fasting however is not only to
abstain from physical food, but also to refrain
from certain feelings, certain thoughts that
weigh us down. Instead of always wanting to absorb, to swallow, accumulate and take too much
of everything, we must learn to renounce, to be
detached. It is this accumulation that makes us
keep going downward. Each thought, each feeling and desire which is not spiritual in nature
weighs us down like frost on the branches of
trees in winter. We need the warm sun of spring
to come and melt the frost so that we can be
again our primordial selves. Once we have rejected all the useless accumulations inside us,
then we will feel ourselves transformed, brought
to life, by the divine breath.

If you keep assimilating things in your head
or heart, you have no room for God and His angels. Do not misunderstand: I am not saying
never to make use of your stomach and lungs
and intestines... no... it is not by destroying your

physical body that you will understand truth. Your body must be intact, head, heart, lungs, stomach and all. The point is for them all to be in harmony: that is the real meaning, the real goal of fasting.

8

HOLY COMMUNION

An essential observance of the Christian church is the sacrament of Holy Communion, although it was not Jesus who founded this institution. Genesis says that centuries before Jesus, Melchisedek, the Priest of the Most High, had come to meet Abraham with the Bread and the Wine.

But communion should not be limited to swallowing from time to time a few wafers that have been blessed by the priest. Each one of us is a High Priest, it is our vocation to come before our cells each day as the officiant bearing them the bread and wine. If you play this role consciously, your cells will receive the real communion from you, that is, the sacred element that will sanctify their work, and the joy they feel in being able to do their work well will reflect on you.

To understand the mystery of the Lord's Supper, you must start with food, with your nourishment. Of course, all the spiritual exercises, breathing, meditation, contemplation, identification, are a form of communion, but in order to understand, you must begin by understanding nutrition. It is not easy for everyone to meditate or contemplate, people may not have the right conditions or opportunity, or even the gift. But everyone eats, they eat every day. The way to understand communion therefore, is to begin on the physical plane.

To communicate is to make an exchange: you give something and you receive something in return. You say that all you do when you eat is take, but you are wrong, you also give something. If you do not, you are not communicating. True communion is a divine exchange. The Holy Eucharist brings you its blessing and benediction but if you take without giving your love and respect, it is not communion, it is dishonest. When you take, you must give. If you give your love and respect, your faith as you partake of the Eucharist, it will give you all of its divine elements. Those who partake of the Holy Eucharist without this holy attitude will never transform themselves, for no object acts on us, it is the confidence and love we put into the object that affects us.

To communicate with God, you must give Him your love, your gratitude, your loyalty. Not that God needs anything you could give Him, He is so tremendously rich that He can do without anything you have, but it is you who, by wanting to give Him something from your heart and soul, awaken certain spiritual centres within, and the divine qualities and virtues begin to flow in abundance.

Now let us come back to nutrition. Even when you are preparing a meal you should be thinking as you touch the food that you are impregnating it with your love. Talk to it, "You who are bringing me life from God, I love you and appreciate you, I know what tremendous wealth there is in you. I have a family, millions and millions of inhabitants inside me to nourish, and so, be kind, give them some of the abundant life you have." If you form the habit of talking this way to your food as you eat it, it will be transformed into strength and light, because you are communicating with Nature. You will see that true communion has a much larger meaning than the Church allows.

Is it intelligent to think that only when you receive the Holy Eucharist are you communicating with God? Besides which, no Eucharist has ever transformed anyone, people swallow wagonloads of wafers and remain the same as before, indolent and morose, with the same tendency to steal and live to excess. Everything depends on whether you are conscious or not that God has put His life into the food you are eating. When you eat it under those conditions you are like the priest who blessed the bread and the wine, and each day, each time you eat, you enter into communication with the divine life.

I believe in understanding and respecting sacred things and that is why I am inviting you to practise these things. I know that the time is coming when each one of us will be a priest before the Eternal. A priest is one who understands God's creation, who loves and honours it and all creatures, whether he is ordained or not. A priest is anyone who is ordained by God. God is above all, He takes orders from no one, He cannot be taken by force and enclosed in a wafer to be distributed to all and sundry. Why try to force God since it is He who enters willingly into our food in the first place? He does not like to be compelled. Often when we think He is there, He is not.

By exaggerating the importance of Holy Communion, humans have neglected the importance of food, our daily nutrition and communion. We have forgotten that it is this food that links us with God. I wish to open your eyes to the fact that the food you eat is as sacred as the Host, because it is nature, which God Himself prepared with His quintessence. Can a priest's blessing add anything to that?

The Church has so misinformed people that now there is no way of making them understand the wonders God has created. What *they* have created, yes, but what God has created... they are above all that. If you question a priest of course he will not say he thinks of himself as superior to God, but in practice it is exactly as if he put himself above Him. Instead of saying, "Respect life, my children, for everything is sacred, everything in Nature is a talisman that God placed there for us," it is only the Church that counts, the Communion, the rosaries, medallions and relics, etc... and nothing else.

I am not diminishing the role of priests, nor am I diminishing the importance of Holy Communion, I want to open new horizons for you, for you to see that Communion is an indispensable act that is to be repeated each day. By communicating two or three times a year, what do you think changes inside you? Nothing, if your cells stay the same you will remain eternally as you are. To change the body, the physical body that is so headstrong, you must work on transforming it every day with all your thought, your love, your faith, and finally, this tough old carcass will begin to vibrate!

The religious rites instituted by the Church

should not assume such importance that they
hide the religion! We often confine ourselves to
a narrow vision of religion and leave all the rest
in the shade. What good does it do if the religion
you belong to hides the splendour of God's creation and keeps humans from turning back to
Him?

9

THE MEANING OF THE BLESSING

Today most of the food we eat has been poisoned by all kinds of chemical products. It is practically impossible to find anything edible that is really fresh, really pure. We grow our fruit and vegetables in fertilizer that is noxious, we catch our fish in polluted waters: how long will humans be able to survive in such a world? Nevertheless, all they seem to care about is their business and profit, and whether we all die of poison or not is of little interest.

It is important for us to know that our food can be affected, altered by our way of thinking about it as we absorb it. The reason for prayer, the purpose of the blessing before meals is to put us in the best possible condition to receive our food. Prayers and blessings cannot add anything to the food in the way of life or vital force, this has already been done by God and His servants, the sun, wind, stars, water, and earth. If we could add life to the food simply by blessing it, why not bless a piece of wood or stone or metal and eat that? No, the blessing cannot add life to the food.

"Then it does no good to bless the food?" you ask. Yes, the words and gestures of the blessing are important because they wrap the food in subtle fluids and emanations that fill whoever eats it with harmony, and his subtle bodies will then be able to accept the riches the food contains.

When two people meet, at first they vibrate differently, it is not always easy to be harmonious at once. As time goes by however, they begin to make exchanges and a sort of osmosis takes place that makes them vibrate in unison. It is the same with food: if you eat thoughtlessly, without preparation, the food remains alien, but if you establish a relation with it ahead of time, it will have an entirely different effect. You have seen how I hold a fruit in my hands before eating it: I do that in order to warm it, to familiarize it with me and make its etheric body open to me and nourish me.

When you want to tame a wild animal, you try first of all to make friends with it, you smile and talk gently to it. Animals, plants, even people, need to feel love before they accept to be tamed! It is the same for food, and also for medicine: you must work on the etheric matter before it can act favourably on your system. A stone in the palm of your hand, if it is made to vibrate in a friendly way becomes protective, it can even heal you. And this law exists in every realm. Take a boy and girl. At first they behave like strangers, the girl sits there, aloof and upright and pure... it is wonderful! But the boy, who is bent on taming her, offers her a drink, he plays sentimental music for her, and soon she capitulates and becomes friendly... tamed!

When you buy a new pair of shoes, at first they are too tight and stiff, you are uncomfortable in them, but little by little they soften and become wearable: they have become used to you. When you move into a new house, a strange room, at first you feel out of place, you are a stranger there. In time it begins to vibrate with you and your life, you enjoy coming back to it : it has become home.

For food it is the same thing. Curiously, no one thinks that food needs to be dealt with in a certain way for a link to be formed between you, for it to be familiarized with you and your needs. Before it is set on your table it has been handled and packed by all kinds of people, transported and stored in all kinds of places, you are strangers, there is no link. But if you pick up a fruit, say, and hold it in your hands lovingly, respectfully, it will begin to vibrate differently, it will become your friend. The secret to making food give the best of itself is to warm it, to fill it with your love before eating it. It will open like a flower and give you its perfume. If you do not like the food before you, do not eat it, for it will be an enemy and your system will be unable to absorb it. Never eat food you dislike.

Now, try this exercise: take a fruit in your hand and mentally talk to it. As you do this, something in the fruit is transformed and when you eat it, it will give you the best of itself and nourish you in all kinds of ways.

There is a power within you that has always been there, it has survived centuries of inertia and stagnation. If you start to do these exercises, to meditate and pray, this power will begin to stir. Concentrate on the desire to add something more to your life, something more subtle and pure than anything you have ever known.

10

THE PURPOSE OF EATING

I

The fruit and vegetables we eat are full of condensed solar energy. We must learn how to extract this energy and send it to the centres for the system to distribute. This can only be done by thinking, by participating in thought as you eat; only by conscious and concentrated thought will you make the food release this imprisoned energy. The process is the same as that in a nuclear centre. Actually, if you knew how to eat, a few mouthfuls would suffice to extract enough energy to stir up the whole universe.

The process of fission is not confined to the stomach alone, it also takes place in the lungs and brain. "In the brain?" you ask. Yes, an Initiate rapt in meditation, in ecstasy, sends out currents and waves and flames into space. Where does all this energy come from? From his brain. And yet the mass weight remains the same. A few particles of matter disintegrate within his brain, and this disintegration releases the psychic energy he sends out into the world.

Our contemporary scientists think it is they who made the discovery of the fission, or the splitting of the atom, but the process has been known to Initiates for thousands of years. They did not reveal their knowledge because of the danger, they knew that man is not yet master of his instincts and that he would use this discovery to destroy the world... which is what is happening. In the future, when humans are more evolved, they will have access to the great mysteries of Nature, they will know how to draw energy from the ocean, the air, the minerals, the trees, etc... and be able to carry out prodigious achievements.

For the moment, it would be enough to realize how much energy there is to be drawn from the food by thinking in a certain way as you eat. Nutrition is no more than a war between the human organism and the matter, the elements to be assimilated: what is acceptable is assimilated, the rest is rejected. For the system to absorb the food properly, it has to tear apart and destroy the food: to build it must first destroy. This is done automatically, unconsciously, but by participating in thought in a certain way, we can work on the food to make it open and permit us to draw the energy we need to accomplish our material and our spiritual work.

II

Man eats, all creatures eat, but why do they eat? Everyone knows why, it is to stay alive. Yes, but is that the only reason? There is more than one reason, one goal, for everything we do, and there is more to eating than merely keeping us alive.

Worms eat the soil, and in so doing they fertilize it; before they eject it they fill it with new qualities. It is the same thing with us and the food we eat. Humans are more highly evolved than matter, or food, they are endowed with life and the power to think and feel, and by making the food pass through their bodies, they transform it into something more alive, more refined, more spiritual.

All creatures, plants, animals, humans, cause the matter they nourish themselves with to evolve, because they impregnate it with new elements. It is the duty of every one of Nature's realms to nourish the realm below it so that it may evolve. This also happens to us, there are beings above, higher and more advanced than we, whose task it is to digest us, that we may be transformed. Life is an uninterrupted series of exchanges between the organic and the inorganic worlds, exchanges that take place on every level. Thus people who are more intelligent educate the ignorant, those who are kind and generous take care of delinquents and criminals, the strong help the weak, the rich give to the poor. Why? For the sake of evolution, for the ones who are behind to evolve. For evolution to take place, there must be an exchange, an exchange between two opposite poles. That is the real reason for eating, the reason behind our need for nutrition. Cosmic Intelligence could no doubt have found some other means of making His creatures evolve, but He chose that one. For each one of His creatures to evolve, he must be absorbed by creatures higher than he, on a plane above his.

I gave you the worm as an example: worms swallow the ground in order to work on it by impregnating it with an element that makes it more alive, and then they eject it. Could it be that humans have the same task, that is, of making matter, the earth, evolve by absorbing it and making it pass through them? You see, men and worms have the same duty, they are collaborators, whether they realize it or not! Before coming down here on earth, they signed contracts promising to work, pledging themselves each in his own way to work on transforming matter in order to vivify it. You are laughing at the idea of a worm signing a contract? Go ahead, laughter is good for you!

The human body is made up of particles of matter that go back when the body dies, into the four elements that formed it: earth, water, air, and fire. If, during man's life here on earth, these particles become more alive and intelligent, more expressive, they will be used to form creatures of a higher order; if the particles have degenerated instead of improving because of the animal or criminal life the body has lived, then they will serve to form only the lower creatures, the grossest and most animal natures. Now do you see how far human responsibility reaches?

Man is responsible during his life on earth and even after his death, for the particles of matter in his body, whether they are impregnated with light, love, kindness and purity, or whether they are impregnated with evil vibrations emanating from egoism, criminal activities, or degenerate living. Even after death he continues to be responsible! He will not be pursued by anyone for the crimes he committed, the debts he incurred, in the world... how could he be caught?

Death solves a lot of problems in the world, but on the other side it is of no help whatsoever, man is held responsible for the evil he left behind, for the effect of his evil thoughts, evil feelings, evil actions. That is the truth, dear brothers and sisters, although most of us are not aware of it and have no idea how far-reaching our responsibility is. To be conscious of one's responsibility is the highest form of consciousness.

Eating, drinking, breathing, working... in everyone of our activities we can transform matter by filling it with what we have, that is, giving it more life, more love, more intelligence and light. Plants nourish themselves on minerals, and in doing so raise them to the plant level; animals eat plants and raise them to the animal level; humans eat animals and raise them to the human level. The question you have never asked is, who eats humans?

Two kinds of creatures nourish themselves on human beings. Just as some people eat, not animals, but animal products such as milk and eggs, etc... so entities in the invisible world eat, not human beings, but their emanations, their thoughts and feelings. Depending upon whether the sustenance you offer is good or bad, that is, lofty thoughts or base thoughts, noble feelings or gross feelings, it serves to nourish either Angels or lower entities. You must understand in which form naturally, but the Angels are food for the Archangels, the Archangels for the Principalities, and so on, all the way up to the Seraphim, whose emanations are food for the Lord.

From earliest times, the Initiates knew that their prodigious Science would be misinterpreted by the uninitiated, the masses, and so they clothed each great truth, each revelation, in imagery to be deciphered by anyone who had sufficient insight. For instance, the Bible says that the Lord delights in the sweet smell of sacrifice and burnt offerings... does this really mean that He takes pleasure in the smell of roasted flesh, or is it not rather an image to show that the spiritual emanations coming from a sacrifice offered to God serve as food for all the higher entities including God Himself? For God also accepts nourishment. Since we are created in His image and we eat, it must be that He also eats. Perhaps not in exactly the same way, with teeth and a stomach and intestines.... God is so pure and so sublime that we cannot imagine Him eating... but would it be mentioned in the Bible if there were not a profound truth hidden behind the image?

Man's task is to absorb matter and enliven it by making it pass through his body. That is the real purpose of eating. Have you any notion how much a man eats in his lifetime? All mankind has been eating for millions of years, and little by little the world has been changing... particularly as there are so many conscientious people, generously doing their work with so much zeal that they even eat lavishly five or six times a day! Contributing to the transformation of matter! The world should reward and encourage such people, yes, for their magnificent work. Think of all the pigs, turkeys, chickens and rabbits that disappear each day thanks to them! Such eagerness to improve the world, such dedication! Whereas the poor vegetarians munching on their meager lettuce leaves, how can you put them on a pedestal? They are way behind the ogres and ogresses!

Actually it is not a question of putting matter only into the stomach, but also of making it pass through the lungs, the heart, the brain. Life does not come to a standstill once we receive it, it goes on flowing forth, and we constantly receive more life, always new, always fresh. Therefore, it is not only by eating that we improve matter, but by our actions, the way we speak, look, walk, work... yes, nutrition embraces all those things too. In order to serve creation, to be useful to the world by putting a divine element into it, even we, we must live a perfect life and be impregnated with light, so that our lives fill everyone and everything around us with light. And then, this ideal of making everything we come in contact with more alive and luminous, more beautiful, that is, transformed, will also transform us. Inside us a total mobilization will take place and the invisible world will join us as our allies, that we may win.

11

THE LAW OF INTERCHANGES

I

It is surprising to note that human beings who pride themselves on knowing the great mysteries of Creation, have completely overlooked such an important process as nutrition, their daily alimentation which God has filled with His love and wisdom. If you were to study the laws of nutrition, you would see that the same laws control all exchanges everywhere in the universe, between the sun and the planets and particularly, in the realm of love. Yes, the law that rules over conception and gestation is the same law that rules over nutrition.

Everything we eat, be it fish or fruit, vegetables or cheese, has a part that needs to be removed before it is edible, either the bones, or the skin, or the crust... in any case, it must be washed and inspected before eating. Such precautions are a necessary precaution to protect your palate, teeth or stomach. Why would it not be the same thing with our psychic nutrition?

Before accepting someone into your heart and soul, should you not make sure they are in a proper condition to be absorbed and digested without causing injury? "But it is love!" you say. Yes I know you think so, but love that is blind is not real love. Real love is enlightened, it is guided by wisdom, not folly.

Most of the time when people meet, they make exchanges, they embrace without any preparation, still covered with the soot accumulated in their heart and soul by passing through the world's chimneys. An Initiate does not do that: when he meets someone, he looks upon that person as a delicious fruit naturally, but like fruit, he must be washed and peeled before eating. That is the difference between the Initiates and ordinary, unenlightened men who make exchanges and associations blindly without using wisdom or knowledge. They are like the cat who swallows the mouse whole, skin and all! And then they complain, "Oh, I am so unhappy with my wife!" or, "Look at what I drew for a husband!" Why act like a cat? Why be in such a hurry to eat that man, that woman, before checking to see what their thinking is, their feeling, their breathing... in other words, their aura?

Now is the time to analyse yourself and, if necessary, to revise your life. You will see that you have always concentrated on details and appearances without looking to see what the person's ideals were, or how they thought and felt about life. Initiates are much harder to please and they are right. They learned the lesson Nature has to teach us about our food, and they apply it to their psychic nutrition as well.

Human beings realize that the food they eat must be gone over and thoroughly cleansed before it is served, but they have not realized that the lesson Nature is trying to teach applies to the psychic plane as well. A mother loves her child more than anything in the world, but if he comes asking to be kissed and hugged after playing in the mud, she will send him to wash himself before kissing him... why not kiss him anyhow if she loves him so much? Dear brothers and sisters, the great Living Book of Nature is spread wide before everyone, but only those who are wise can interpret it.

You will go to immense trouble selecting the food you eat three times a day, making sure it is good... but you will accept anyone that comes along in your life, regardless. As a result, your life is poisoned. God is the only one you can love without bothering to know Him. You never will know God unless you love Him, and the same is true for a great Master: unless you begin by loving him, he will remain closed. But humans need to be known before you love them, that is, before eating them, or accepting them into your inner sanctuary.

The question is how to love a Master. People are apt to think of a Master as a lake in which they can wash and get rid of their dirt, never thinking that other people drink the water in that lake, and what will be left for them? People come to see a Master to pour out all the filth they have picked up during their lives, leaving it to him to wash them of their impurity, or transform it, thus adding to his already overloaded schedule. If a Master feels the need to purify himself, shouldn't other people? Ah, they think they are spotless, they can't see the filth the devils and demons they have been with have left on them.

But let us leave all that and come back to the lesson to be drawn from eating food. People are like fruit or any other food, in that they have one part that is not digestible and one that is delicious and tasty. That is the one to preserve. Each one of us has a spark inside, put there by God, and it is that spark that you should look for in each other. If you look at the spark instead of merely at the external side, you will find that everyone and everything has it, animals, plants, stones... even criminals. And if you can animate that spark, by addressing yourself to it, you will be able to communicate with the whole world, even with criminals.

Initiates do not choose to relate to man's lower nature, his personality; knowing that rats and such things live in the cellar, they prefer to remain above on the higher levels. Unlike other people who are interested in each other's defects and spend their time talking about that when they meet, an Initiate seeks the buried spark in others, in order to link them to the Heavenly Father and the Divine Mother. He works on people in that way, and one day, the light comes and they are flooded with it, thanks to the work he has done. In that way a Master works to improve his disciples, always addressing himself only to the divine spark in each one. For that reason they love him and allow him to draw out the best in them.

You too when you meet someone, should think about discovering the divine spark hidden within, his Higher Self, for in that way you help him to form a link with God. That is love in its highest, most evolved form, to be able to connect with the divine spark in each creature and feed and strengthen it. There is no need to be on one's guard if you do that, no need to waste time studying the person before allowing yourself to love and accept him, because the spark is entirely pure. Whereas, if it is a question of his personality, it is better to know before accepting it. The divine spark that shines within each one can always be accepted instantly without hesitation.

II

If you look upon human beings as fruit, as I suggested, you will find when you are looking at them, listening to them and talking with them, that you can in fact, taste them. Usually you see only the outside, the clothes they are wearing, the jewels, their face and hair, but not the hidden life of their soul and spirit. Actually that is all that should interest you. Instead, you stop short at the impression, the surface, you take snapshots, "Ah, there's a girl I would like to sleep with!" What do you know of her? Her legs, her pretty figure, her little turned up nose: your interest is limited to your own desire for amusement and satisfaction.

An Initiate likes to eat, but he prefers divine food, he looks for the divine life in people. When he finds fruit and flowers, that is, humans who vibrate with divine life, then he is happy, content to admire their beautiful forms and colours and breathe their emanations, he does not need to devour them. Nevertheless, he is satisfied, because this fruit, these flowers, have brought him closer to Heaven.

If you can understand nutrition, real nutrition, you will see that it solves all problems, including sex. Yes, anyone who has decided not to touch food at all, that is, to avoid men or women because it is supposedly the way to be pure and chaste, is on his way to spiritual death, perhaps even physical death. You can eat everything once you know in what way to eat.

The secret lies in taking homeopathic doses, that is confining oneself to looking, listening, breathing. You will never become a saint by giving up eating, you will never know anything at all that way, least of all God. Life will abandon you if you do that, you will have no inspiration, no verve, no joy. Sainthood is itself nutrition, dear brothers and sisters, that is the Initiatic way of looking at it. Instead of eating impure, dense food, saints eat divine food. In the realm of sexuality, humans always go to extremes, they either starve themselves to death, or they are gluttons.

When you start to study nutrition, you will see that there are different ways of eating on every one of the planes. You will see that it is not possible to live without eating, and even the Angels, even God Himself, must eat. God eats

the subtle quintessence from the trees He plant-
ed: His creatures. Yes, God eats and is in good
health, I promise you, because He never absorbs
impurity. He leaves it to others to transform
their impurity before offering themselves to
Him.

You ask how it is possible to tell the difference between someone who eats in the right way
and someone who does not? Is it not easy to see
the difference between the beggar who scrounges
for food in garbage cans and the prince who sits
down every day to a table laden with delicious
dishes? In the spiritual world it is the same: Initiates have another bearing, another demeanour
that distinguishes them from average men, prov-
ing that they are well 'fed,' whereas the average
man pays no attention to what he eats.

My criterion is that when I see someone
whose face has no light, I know at once that he is
undernourished. You say, "Well, but he goes to
church, he gives to the poor, he lowers his eyes
in the presence of women...." Possibly. Nevertheless, I can see that inside he prefers gamy,
decadent food, that is what he likes. When I
meet someone who radiates with light, no matter
what I am told about him, I think, "I wonder
what his secret is, he is like a spring that flows!"
You say, "But I saw him staring at the girls on
the beach!" That is not important, the impor-

tant thing is what he sees, how he looks at them.

If someone receives a lift toward God as a result of his admiration and wonderment whenever he sees feminine beauty, why interfere? "But someone who is pure, a saint, would never look that way, it goes against all the traditional rules." Well, then, tell me why you, for all your purity and saintliness, are weak and drab, without any light, inspiration or enthusiasm? Is that what saintliness does for you? And why does that fellow, in spite of his staring at women, radiate with all the light and glory of Heaven? This is something to think about. You see how true it is that humans do not know how to think!

Exchanges form the basis of life, the exchanges we make with food, with water and air, with our fellow humans and other creatures in the universe, with Angels and Archangels, and with God. It is not only when we eat and drink that we make exchanges, or rather, yes, it is when we eat and drink that we make exchanges that bring us life, that keep us alive on all planes, not only on the physical plane. When I say that nutrition comes first and is more important that anything, I am speaking of nutrition on every plane, the food we eat and the exchanges we make in all the regions of the universe that nourish the whole man, not only the physical body, but all the subtle bodies also. If I am always insisting on the need for psychic purification as well as physical purification, it is because purity re-establishes communication, and once communication with the higher regions is restored, you receive the luminous currents of energy that circulate in space.

Prayer, meditation, contemplation, ecstasy and rapture, are all forms of nutrition, glorious nutrition called celestial ambrosia. Every religion speaks of this immortal beverage that the Alchemists called the Elixir of Eternal Life. This Elixir can be tasted on the physical plane, but only on one condition : that you go and find it in the purest and highest regions.

Our reason for contemplating the sunrise is to drink this ambrosia that the sun distributes so generously on rocks, plants, animals, humans, and all creation. Plants are more intelligent than humans, they know that if they link themselves with the sun, there will be results. Humans prefer to sleep until noon, or watch the sunset, they are not drawn to something that climbs and expands and flowers, but prefer things that are falling, dying, vanishing. The law says that you eventually resemble what you look at and admire, and so by concentrating on the setting sun, you become inwardly feebler and feebler until you become extinguished.

You will find that the meaning of life is hidden in nutrition, if your food is the pure, shining particles, the celestial, eternal quintessences that are found in the sun. By concentrating on the sun each morning and trying to breathe in its quintessence, your health will improve, you will become bright and radiant, with a strong will and a joyful heart.

You say you have been going to the sunrise for years and have never noticed anything. That is because you do not know how to look at the sun. It is the way in which you do things, the intense love and thought that you put into it that bring results... not the amount of time you devote. Whenever you feel alive and fulfilled, like today for instance, it is because you have drawn a few draughts of life at the source, the inexhaustible spring of the sun. Is it so difficult to understand?

The sun is nutrition, dear brothers and sisters, never forget that, it is the best food of all. Why be limited to the elements of earth, water, and air? There is another element and we must learn to nourish ourselves with it: fire, the light. That is what we do at sunrise.

When Zoroaster asked Ahura Mazda what the first man nourished himself with, Ahura Mazda replied, "He ate the fire and he drank the light," meaning that he was nurtured by the sun's rays, he received life from the sun, and thus was able to understand the Mysteries of the universe.

III

If I were to tell you that the laws governing nutrition are the same as the laws that govern conception, you would be surprised and probably not see any connection. There is a connection, for the minute you sit down to eat, you are creating conditions that will affect the birth of thoughts and feelings and actions. You cannot create without eating. The condition the mother and father are in during the conception of a child, determines the child's destiny; the state you are in when you eat, determines the nature of your physical and psychic comportment. Each mouthful of food is a conception. What is your state of mind whilst you are conceiving?

Food is the living seed that produces a child, that is, the child of your thinking, feeling, acting. What are the forces that will be the issue of your union? Will the children be misshapen weaklings because of their parents' ignorance? It is you who are the father, since you contribute the food, and your physical body is the mother: if neither mother nor father is intelligent, attentive, reasonable and sound of mind and body, the result will be catastrophic.

When you eat in a state of anger, discontent or distress before leaving for work, say, you will be upset all day, your vibrations will be chaotic, and everything you do will be affected. Even if you appear calm, your emanations will betray your inner agitation and tension, no matter how you try to control them. Whereas if you eat in harmonious conditions, you will remain harmonious all day, no matter how much you have to run around, or how much stress you are under, peace will be inside you and it will not be dislodged.

Do not take your anxiety and problems to the table with you, leave them outside the door, to be resumed when you have finished eating if you must. If you eat harmoniously, it gives you the solution to your problems. I repeat, meals are an opportunity for spiritual exercise : begin by clearing your mind of anything that might keep you from eating peacefully and in harmony, and if you cannot manage peace at once, wait until you calm down, for otherwise you will only poison your system, the food will be contaminated by your anxiety and you will be in a chaotic state... the result of eating under the wrong conditions.

But how will humans ever understand the importance of the state they are in when they eat, if they cannot create a child (an act that is even more consequential) without hating each other? Have they any idea what dreadful things they give their child-to-be that way, how much he will suffer as a result? And then he in turn will be filled with poison, and pour it out on everyone around him.

Nutrition is a form of conception, and love is a form of nutrition. Heaven will hold you responsible, you know, for what you put into the heart and soul of your partner. The rest is a matter of indifference. But if you embrace your beloved when you are unhappy and discouraged, to make yourself feel better (a frequent occurrence), you are doing something that is criminal: contaminating the other person with all your misery and filth. You should not choose that moment. Love anyone you like, kiss anyone you like, but not before you have made sure in your heart and soul that you are giving them nothing but love and light. Under those conditions Heaven will condone your action. Humans may condemn you for it, but Heaven will be applauding.

A child spends nine months in his mother's womb and when he is born, his umbilical cord is cut and he is left to nourish himself independently. It is true that he is no longer in his mother's womb, but he is in the womb of another mother, Mother Nature, and is nourished through another umbilical cord, the solar plexus. In countries such as India, China, Japan, there exist ancient techniques for nourishing yourself through the solar plexus. You would like me to describe those techniques, I know, but what good will it do if you cannot even eat in the right spirit?

It is impossible not to be filled with admiration for the beautiful way in which Divine Intelligence has arranged things. By the simple gesture of eating a fruit, you put life in your entire organism! Divine Intelligence has known what each organ, each cell, each little atom in our bodies needs, to make the whole go on living! Thanks to the food we eat, we go on seeing, hearing, breathing, tasting, touching, speaking, singing, walking... and our hair, nails, teeth, skin, etc... all receive exactly what they need in order to keep growing. Yes, one cannot possibly not be lost in wonder and admiration.

From now on, you should think a little more often about linking yourself with this Intelligence, about showing your gratitude. You might ask to be allowed to assist Nature in the work, and then when you are ready, you will be ac-

cepted in the various working sites and shown
how to work, either on yourself, or down in the
bowels of the earth on minerals, metals, crystals
and precious stones. You will make extraordinary discoveries.

Where do you suppose this Initiatic Science
originated? It was given to mankind by the
higher Beings who were able to develop the fac-
ulty of bilocation, and were thus enabled to visit
the centre of the earth, the depths of the ocean,
the other planets, and even the sun! They wit-
nessed the unimaginable land, peopled with
highly evolved, luminous creatures, the *"Aretz
ha Haim"* of the Psalms, the Land of the Living,
which is the sun.

These highly evolved Spirits left us the Initiatic Science as our heritage, and it is this
Science, this Heritage, that I am now presenting
to you. Let me quickly say that I too know very
little about it, but I trust in time to know
more.... Do not, I beseech you, take this hope
from me!

Distributed by:

BELGIUM: Mrs Brigitte VAN MEERBEECK
Chemin du Gros Tienne, 112
B - 1328 Lasne-Ohain

BRITISH ISLES: PROSVETA Ltd.
4 St Helena Terrace
Richmond, Surrey TW9 1NR

Trade orders to:
ELEMENT Books Ltd
The Old Brewery, Tilsbury, Salisbury
Wiltshire SP3 6NH

CANADA: PROSVETA Inc. - 1565 Montée Masson
Duvernay est, Laval
Que. H7E 4P2

FRANCE: Editions PROSVETA S.A. - B.P. 12
83601 Fréjus Cedex

GERMANY: URANIA
Steindorfstraße 14
D - 8000 München 22

GREECE: PROSVETA GRÈCE
90, Bd. Vassileos Constantinou
Le Pirée

ITALY: PROSVETA
Bastelli 7
I - 43036 Fidenza (Parma)

PORTUGAL: Ediçãoes Idade d'Ouro
Rua Passos Manuel 20 – 3.° Esq.
P - 1100 Lisboa

SPAIN: PROSVETA ESPAÑOLA
Caspe 41
Barcelona-10

SWITZERLAND: PROSVETA Société Coopérative
CH - 1801 Les Monts-de-Corsier

UNITED-STATES: PROSVETA U.S.A.
P.O. Box 49614 Los Angeles
California 90049

Any enquiries should be addressed to the nearest distributor

NOTES